PLANT-BASED DIET COOKBOOK

Delicious Recipes For Every Meal: A Comprehensive Guide To Mastering Plant-Based Eating, Including Breakfasts, Lunches, Dinners, Snacks, And Desserts

Charlotte Harry

Table of Contents

CHAPTER ONE

INTRODUCTION TO PLANT-BASED EATING

What Is A Plant-Based Diet?

A plant-based diet primarily focuses on foods derived from plants. This includes not only fruits and vegetables but also nuts, seeds, oils, whole grains, legumes, and beans. A common misconception is that a plant-based diet means being vegetarian or vegan and entirely giving up meat or animal products. However, this is not necessarily the case. Instead, a plant-based diet means proportionately choosing more of your foods from plant sources. This approach emphasizes whole, minimally processed plant foods and can vary greatly depending on individual choices, cultural traditions, and nutritional needs.

A plant-based diet does not strictly exclude meat or animal products. Many people following a plant-based diet may still incorporate small amounts of meat or dairy into their meals. The primary focus is on increasing the intake of plant foods, which are rich in essential nutrients, fiber, and antioxidants. This dietary pattern can provide numerous health benefits, including a lower risk of chronic diseases such as heart disease, diabetes, and certain cancers.

One of the key aspects of a plant-based diet is its flexibility. Individuals can adapt their eating habits based on personal preferences and health goals. For example, someone might choose to follow a strict vegan diet, avoiding all animal products, while others might opt for a more flexible approach, including occasional servings of meat or dairy. The emphasis is on making plant foods the central part of the diet rather than the exclusion of animal products entirely.

Cultural traditions also play a significant role in shaping plant-based diets. In many cultures, plant-based eating has been a long-standing tradition. For instance, the Mediterranean diet, which includes a high intake of fruits, vegetables, nuts, and olive oil, has been associated with numerous health benefits. Similarly, traditional Asian diets often emphasize rice, vegetables, and legumes, with meat consumed in smaller quantities.

Nutritional needs are another important consideration when adopting a plant-based diet. It is essential to ensure that the diet provides all necessary nutrients, including protein, iron, calcium, and vitamin B12, which are often associated with animal products. Fortunately, plant-based diets can meet these nutritional needs with careful planning and the inclusion of a variety of foods. For instance, legumes, nuts, seeds, and whole grains are excellent sources of protein, while leafy greens and fortified plant milks can provide calcium.

Benefits Of Plant-Based Eating

Adopting a plant-based diet offers numerous health benefits, significantly impacting both personal well-being and the environment. A primary advantage of plant-based eating is its potential to reduce the risk of chronic diseases. Extensive research has shown that such diets can lower the incidence of heart disease, high blood pressure, diabetes, and certain types of cancer. This is largely due to the fact that plant-based diets are typically low in saturated fats and cholesterol while being high in dietary fiber. The high fiber content promotes better heart health and aids in maintaining optimal digestive function, thus contributing to overall health improvement.

Weight management is another notable benefit of a plant-based diet. Foods derived from plants generally have a lower calorie density compared to animal products, which means they provide fewer calories per gram while being rich in essential nutrients. This characteristic can lead to weight loss or make it easier to maintain a healthy weight without the need for stringent calorie counting. The high nutrient density of plant foods ensures that the body receives adequate vitamins, minerals, and other vital compounds, supporting various bodily functions and enhancing overall vitality.

Energy levels can also see a significant boost with a plant-based diet. Whole plant foods are rich in essential nutrients, including vitamins, minerals, and antioxidants, that play crucial roles in maintaining energy levels and promoting overall well-being. These nutrients support the body's immune health, helping to ward off illnesses and keep the body functioning optimally. Many people who switch to a plant-based diet report feeling more energized and experiencing improved mood and mental clarity.

Beyond individual health benefits, plant-based eating also promotes environmental sustainability. The production of plant foods generally requires fewer natural resources, such as water and land, and results in lower greenhouse gas emissions compared to animal farming. This reduction in resource usage and emissions helps mitigate the impact of climate change and preserve natural ecosystems. By choosing a plant-based diet, individuals can significantly reduce their carbon footprint, contributing to a more sustainable and healthier planet.

Ethical considerations also play a vital role in the appeal of plant-based eating. Reducing the consumption of animal products decreases the demand for factory-farmed animal products, which often involve practices that raise ethical concerns regarding animal welfare. A plant-based diet supports more humane treatment of animals, aligning with values of compassion and ethical responsibility.

Common Myths And Misconceptions

Despite its numerous benefits, plant-based eating is often surrounded by myths and misconceptions. A prevalent myth is the belief that a plant-based diet cannot provide sufficient protein. This misconception persists despite the availability of numerous plant-based protein sources. Beans, lentils, tofu, tempeh, quinoa, nuts, and seeds are all excellent sources of protein. These foods can easily meet the protein needs of individuals, including athletes and bodybuilders, when consumed in appropriate quantities and combinations.

Another common misconception is that plant-based diets are prohibitively expensive. While it is true that some specialty vegan products can be pricey, a diet that focuses on whole grains, legumes, and seasonal produce can be very cost-effective. Staples like rice, beans, oats, and potatoes are some of the most affordable and nutritious foods available. By planning meals around these economical options and buying in bulk, individuals can maintain a plant-based diet without straining their budgets. Moreover, seasonal fruits and vegetables often cost less and can add variety and nutrition to meals.

A belief that plant-based diets are restrictive and monotonous also persists. This couldn't be further from the truth. Plant-based eating opens up a world of culinary possibilities. There is a vast array of fruits, vegetables, grains, and legumes from different cultures that can make meals exciting and diverse. Exploring cuisines from around the world, such as Mediterranean, Indian, Middle Eastern, and Southeast Asian, can introduce a variety of flavors and ingredients that may not have been previously considered. Far from being limited, plant-based diets encourage creativity and experimentation in the kitchen.

Many people also think that transitioning to a plant-based diet is challenging and requires giving up their favorite foods. In reality, there are numerous delicious plant-based alternatives and recipes that can replicate the flavors and textures of traditional dishes. For instance, there are plant-based versions of burgers, pizzas, ice creams, and even cheeses. These alternatives are becoming increasingly accessible and can make the transition smoother and more enjoyable. Additionally, the growing availability of plant-based products in supermarkets and restaurants has made it easier than ever to find satisfying and familiar foods that fit within a plant-based framework.

Transitioning To A Plant-Based Diet

Transitioning to a plant-based diet can be a gradual and enjoyable journey that doesn't require an overnight overhaul of your eating habits. A practical approach is to start small, incorporating more plant-based meals into your weekly routine. For instance, you could adopt "Meatless Mondays," dedicating one day a week to plant-based eating. Gradually, you can increase the number of plant-based meals, experimenting with replacing meat in your favorite dishes with plant-based proteins like beans, lentils, or tofu. This step-by-step approach allows your palate to adjust and helps you discover new, delicious plant-based recipes.

One of the keys to a successful transition is planning balanced meals that ensure you're getting all the necessary nutrients. While plant-based diets can provide a wealth of health benefits, it's essential to pay close attention to specific nutrients that are sometimes less abundant in plant foods.

Protein, for example, can be sourced from a variety of plant-based foods such as legumes, nuts, seeds, and whole grains. Iron, another crucial nutrient, can be found in foods like spinach, lentils, and chickpeas. Combining these with vitamin C-rich foods like citrus fruits can enhance iron absorption.

Calcium, traditionally associated with dairy products, is also found in plant-based sources such as fortified plant milks, tofu, and leafy green vegetables like kale and bok choy. Vitamin B12, which is primarily found in animal products, may require supplementation or consumption of fortified foods like nutritional yeast and plant-based milks. Omega-3 fatty acids, essential for heart and brain health, can be obtained from flaxseeds, chia seeds, walnuts, and algae-based supplements.

To ease the transition, it can be helpful to find a community or support group. Many online forums, local meet-ups, and social media groups are dedicated to plant-based eating and can offer advice, share recipes, and provide encouragement. Engaging with a supportive community can make the process more enjoyable and less daunting.

Exploring new recipes and experimenting with different fruits, vegetables, grains, and legumes can make the transition exciting and delicious. The variety in plant-based foods is vast, offering endless possibilities for flavorful and nutritious meals. By gradually incorporating these foods into your diet, you can develop a sustainable and enjoyable plant-based eating pattern

that meets your nutritional needs and
supports your overall health and well-being.

CHAPTER TWO

ESSENTIAL NUTRIENTS AND INGREDIENTS

Key Nutrients In A Plant-Based Diet

A plant-based diet is celebrated for its abundant supply of nutrients essential for maintaining optimal health. These nutrients, including vitamins, minerals, fiber, and antioxidants, play pivotal roles in promoting overall well-being and preventing various chronic diseases. Key nutrients to emphasize in a plant-based diet are protein, healthy fats, vitamins, and minerals. Understanding these nutrients and their sources is fundamental to creating a balanced and nutritious diet.

Protein is a critical component of a plant-based diet, necessary for building and repairing tissues, producing enzymes and hormones, and supporting immune function. Contrary to common misconceptions, plant-based diets can provide adequate protein through a variety of sources. Legumes, such as beans, lentils, and chickpeas, are excellent sources of protein. Additionally, nuts, seeds, and whole grains like quinoa and brown rice contribute significantly to protein intake. Incorporating a diverse array of these foods ensures a complete amino acid profile, crucial for optimal health.

Healthy fats are another essential element of a plant-based diet. These fats support brain function, hormone production, and the absorption of fat-soluble vitamins. Sources of healthy fats in a plant-based diet include avocados, nuts, seeds, and plant oils such as olive oil and flaxseed oil. Omega-3 fatty acids, vital for heart health, can be obtained from flaxseeds, chia seeds, hemp seeds, and walnuts. Including these fats in your diet can help reduce inflammation and support overall cardiovascular health.

Vitamins are indispensable for various bodily functions, and a plant-based diet can provide an abundant supply of these essential nutrients. Vitamin C, found in citrus fruits, bell peppers, and leafy greens, is crucial for immune function and skin health. B vitamins, necessary for energy production and brain health, are abundant in whole grains, legumes, nuts, and seeds. Vitamin A, important for vision and immune function, is present in orange and yellow vegetables like carrots, sweet potatoes, and pumpkins. For those following a strict plant-based diet, vitamin B12 supplementation might be necessary, as it is primarily found in animal products.

Minerals such as iron, calcium, magnesium, and zinc are vital for maintaining various bodily functions. Leafy greens, legumes, nuts, seeds, and whole grains are excellent sources of these minerals. Iron, essential for oxygen transport in the blood, can be found in lentils, chickpeas, and fortified cereals. Calcium, crucial for bone health, is abundant in leafy greens, tofu, and fortified plant milks. Magnesium, involved in over 300 biochemical reactions in the body, is present in nuts, seeds, and whole grains. Zinc, important for immune function and wound healing, can be obtained from legumes, nuts, and seeds.

Fiber, a key component of plant-based diets, is vital for digestive health. It aids in maintaining regular bowel movements, reducing cholesterol levels, and stabilizing blood sugar levels. Fruits, vegetables, whole grains, legumes, nuts, and seeds are all excellent sources of dietary fiber. A diet rich in fiber supports a healthy gut microbiome, which is crucial for overall health and well-being.

Plant-Based Protein Sources

Protein is a crucial nutrient that plays a vital role in muscle repair, immune function, and overall growth. While many people traditionally associate protein with animal products, numerous plant-based sources can provide adequate amounts of this essential nutrient. These plant-based proteins are not only rich in protein but also offer a range of additional health benefits, making them a valuable component of a balanced diet.

One of the most well-known and versatile plant-based protein sources is legumes. This category includes beans, lentils, and chickpeas, all of which are excellent sources of both protein and fiber. Legumes are incredibly versatile in the kitchen and can be used in a wide variety of dishes, from soups and stews to salads and spreads. For example, black beans can be added to tacos, while chickpeas can be blended into a creamy hummus. Lentils, with their quick cooking time, make a hearty addition to soups and curries. The high fiber content in legumes also aids in digestion and helps maintain a healthy gut.

Tofu and tempeh are another popular choice for those seeking plant-based protein. Both are made from soybeans, but they differ in texture and preparation. Tofu is smooth and can be used in both savory and sweet dishes, making it incredibly versatile. It can be stir-fried, grilled, blended into smoothies, or even used as a base for vegan desserts. Tempeh, on the other hand, is fermented and has a firmer texture, making it an excellent meat substitute in dishes like stir-fries and sandwiches. The fermentation process also adds beneficial probiotics, which support gut health.

Quinoa is an ancient grain that has gained popularity in recent years due to its high protein content and status as a complete protein. This means it contains all nine essential amino acids that our bodies cannot produce on their own. Quinoa is not only a great source of protein but also rich in fiber, magnesium, and iron. It can be used as a base for salads, served as a side dish, or incorporated into breakfast bowls for a nutritious start to the day.

Nuts and seeds are another powerhouse of plant-based protein. Almonds, chia seeds, hemp seeds, and sunflower seeds are all high in protein and healthy fats. They can be easily added to smoothies, oatmeal, or yogurt for a protein boost. Almonds can also be turned into almond butter, which makes a delicious and protein-rich spread for toast or fruit. Chia seeds and hemp seeds can be sprinkled on top of salads or blended into dressings for added texture and nutrition.

Whole grains such as brown rice, oats, and barley also offer a decent amount of protein along with additional nutrients like fiber, vitamins, and minerals. These grains can be used as a base for many meals, providing sustained energy and keeping you full longer. For instance, oats make a hearty breakfast option, while brown rice and barley can be used in a variety of savory dishes.

Essential Fats And Omega-3s

Healthy fats are a crucial component of a well-balanced diet, playing vital roles in brain function, hormone production, and the structural integrity of cells. While it is advisable to limit the intake of saturated and trans fats due to their association with health issues, unsaturated fats, especially omega-3 fatty acids, are indispensable for maintaining good health.

Plant-based sources of healthy fats are diverse and include avocados, nuts, seeds, and various oils. Avocados are a particularly rich source of monounsaturated fats, which are known to be heart-healthy. These fats help reduce bad cholesterol levels in the bloodstream, thereby lowering the risk of heart disease and stroke. The creamy texture of avocados makes them a versatile ingredient in salads, spreads, and even smoothies, contributing both nutritional value and delicious flavor.

Nuts and seeds are another excellent source of healthy fats. Walnuts, flaxseeds, and chia seeds are particularly high in omega-3 fatty acids, a type of polyunsaturated fat that is essential for the body. Omega-3 fatty acids play a significant role in reducing inflammation, which is a common underlying factor in many chronic diseases, including heart disease and arthritis. Additionally, they support cardiovascular health by improving the balance of fats in the blood and promoting healthy blood vessels. Including a handful of nuts or a sprinkle of seeds in your daily diet can make a significant difference in your omega-3 intake.

Olive oil, widely celebrated for its health benefits, is a staple in many plant-based diets. It is a good source of monounsaturated fats and contains antioxidants that contribute to overall health. Regular consumption of olive oil has been linked to a lower risk of chronic diseases, including heart disease and cancer. Its versatility in cooking, from salad dressings to sautéing vegetables, makes it an easy addition to any diet.

Coconut oil, though often debated, contains medium-chain triglycerides (MCTs), which can be beneficial when consumed in moderation. MCTs are metabolized differently from other fats, providing a quick source of energy and potentially aiding in weight management. However, due to its high saturated fat content, it is important to use coconut oil sparingly within a balanced diet.

Omega-3 fatty acids are particularly noteworthy for their health benefits. They are crucial in managing inflammation and supporting cardiovascular health. Plant-based sources of omega-3s include flaxseeds, chia seeds, hemp seeds, and walnuts. These foods are easily incorporated into various meals—flaxseeds and chia seeds can be added to smoothies, oatmeal, or baked goods, while hemp seeds and walnuts can enhance the nutritional profile of salads and snacks.

Incorporating these healthy fats into a plant-based diet is essential for maintaining optimal health. By choosing a variety of sources, such as avocados, nuts, seeds, olive oil, and coconut oil, you can ensure that you are getting a good balance of essential fats, including the all-important omega-3 fatty acids.

A plant-based diet can provide a comprehensive array of vitamins and minerals necessary for optimal health. However, it is crucial to be mindful of certain nutrients that might require extra attention to ensure they are adequately included in the diet. These nutrients include Vitamin B12, iron, calcium, Vitamin D, zinc, and iodine.

Vitamin B12 is a vital nutrient primarily found in animal products. It plays a key role in maintaining healthy nerve cells and producing DNA. For individuals following a plant-based diet, obtaining sufficient Vitamin B12 can be challenging. Therefore, vegans should consider incorporating fortified foods, such as plant-based milks and breakfast cereals, or taking B12 supplements to meet their daily requirements. Regular monitoring of B12 levels can also help in preventing deficiencies.

Iron is another essential nutrient that requires attention in a plant-based diet. Iron is crucial for transporting oxygen throughout the body and supporting overall energy levels. While plant-based sources of iron, such as lentils, chickpeas, tofu, and spinach, are available, they contain non-heme iron, which is less readily absorbed by the body compared to heme iron found in animal products. To enhance iron absorption, it is beneficial to pair iron-rich foods with vitamin C-rich foods, such as bell peppers, citrus fruits, and tomatoes. This combination can significantly boost iron absorption and prevent iron-deficiency anemia.

Calcium is essential for maintaining strong bones and teeth, as well as supporting muscle function and nerve signaling. While dairy products are well-known sources of calcium, plant-based alternatives can also provide adequate amounts. Fortified plant milks, such as almond, soy, and oat milk, are excellent sources of calcium. Additionally, tofu, almonds, sesame seeds, and leafy greens like kale and broccoli are rich in calcium and can be included in a balanced plant-based diet.

Vitamin D plays a crucial role in bone health by aiding calcium absorption. It can be obtained through sunlight exposure, but in areas with limited sunlight or during winter months, supplementation may be necessary. Fortified foods, such as plant-based milks and cereals, can also provide a source of Vitamin D. Regularly checking Vitamin D levels and considering supplements can help maintain optimal bone health.

Zinc is important for immune function, wound healing, and DNA synthesis. Plant-based sources of zinc include beans, lentils, tofu, and seeds like pumpkin and sunflower seeds. Including a variety of these foods in the diet can help meet zinc requirements. Additionally, soaking and sprouting legumes and seeds can enhance zinc absorption.

Iodine is essential for thyroid function and maintaining a healthy metabolism. While iodine is commonly found in seafood and dairy products, plant-based sources are limited. Iodized salt and seaweed are excellent sources of iodine for individuals following a plant-based diet. Incorporating these into meals can help ensure adequate iodine intake and prevent thyroid-related issues.

Stocking A Plant-Based Pantry

Stocking a well-equipped pantry is crucial for anyone following a plant-based diet. This ensures that you always have the necessary ingredients on hand to prepare nutritious and satisfying meals. A well-stocked pantry can make meal preparation more convenient, enjoyable, and versatile. Here are some essential items to include:

Grains form the foundation of many plant-based meals, providing essential nutrients and serving as a versatile base for various dishes. Brown rice, quinoa, oats, barley, and whole wheat pasta are excellent choices. Brown rice and quinoa are rich in fiber and protein, making them ideal for salads, stir-fries, and grain bowls. Oats can be used for breakfast, snacks, or baking, while barley adds a hearty touch to soups and stews. Whole wheat pasta is a nutritious alternative to regular pasta and can be used in a variety of dishes.

Legumes are a staple in plant-based diets due to their high protein and fiber content. Canned or dried beans, lentils, chickpeas, and peas are essential pantry items. Beans, such as black beans, kidney beans, and navy beans, are versatile and can be used in soups, stews, salads, and burritos. Lentils cook quickly and are perfect for soups, curries, and salads. Chickpeas can be roasted for snacks, mashed for spreads, or used in stews and salads. Peas are great for adding to soups, stews, and pasta dishes.

Nuts and seeds provide healthy fats, protein, and essential nutrients. Almonds, walnuts, chia seeds, flaxseeds, and sunflower seeds are excellent additions to a plant-based pantry. Almonds and walnuts can be used for snacking, baking, or adding to salads and grain bowls. Chia seeds and flaxseeds are rich in omega-3 fatty acids and can be added to smoothies, oatmeal, and baked goods. Sunflower seeds are great for snacking or adding to salads and trail mixes.

Nut butters offer a convenient and tasty source of healthy fats and protein. Peanut butter, almond butter, and tahini are versatile options. They can be used as spreads, added to smoothies, or incorporated into sauces and dressings. Tahini, made from sesame seeds, is a key ingredient in hummus and can also be used in salad dressings and dips.

Plant-based milks are essential for those avoiding dairy. Almond milk, soy milk, oat milk, and coconut milk are popular choices. These can be used in cooking, baking, smoothies, and as a beverage. Soy milk is high in protein, making it a good choice for coffee and tea, while almond and oat milk are great for cereals and smoothies.

Canned goods provide convenience and a long shelf life. Tomatoes, tomato paste, coconut milk, and vegetable broth are must-haves. Canned tomatoes and tomato paste are essential for sauces, soups, and stews. Coconut milk adds richness to curries and soups, while vegetable broth serves as a base for soups and stews.

Spices and herbs enhance the flavor of plant-based dishes. Turmeric, cumin, paprika, basil, oregano, and thyme are versatile and can be used in a variety of recipes. Turmeric and cumin add warmth and depth to curries and stews, while paprika, basil, oregano, and thyme are perfect for seasoning pasta sauces, soups, and roasted vegetables.

Oils and vinegars are crucial for cooking and dressing salads. Olive oil, coconut oil, apple cider vinegar, and balsamic vinegar are essential pantry staples. Olive oil is great for sautéing and salad dressings, while coconut oil is ideal for baking and stir-frying. Apple cider vinegar and balsamic vinegar add acidity and depth to salads and marinades.

Snacks are important for maintaining energy levels between meals. Dried fruits, whole grain crackers, and dark chocolate are nutritious and satisfying options. Dried fruits provide a natural sweetness and can be added to trail mixes or eaten on their own. Whole grain crackers are perfect for pairing with nut butters or hummus, and dark chocolate offers a delicious treat with health benefits.

CHAPTER THREE

BREAKFAST RECIPES

Smoothies And Smoothie Bowls

Starting your day with a nutrient-packed breakfast is essential for maintaining energy levels and overall health, and what better way to achieve this than with smoothies and smoothie bowls? These breakfast options are not only delicious but also incredibly versatile and easy to make. By blending a variety of fruits, vegetables, nuts, and seeds, you can create a meal that is both satisfying and nourishing.

A basic smoothie can be as simple as combining bananas, berries, and spinach with a liquid base like almond milk or coconut water. Bananas provide a natural sweetness and a creamy texture, while berries add a burst of flavor and antioxidants. Spinach, although mild in taste, is a powerhouse of nutrients, including vitamins A, C, and K, as well as folate and iron. Using almond milk or coconut water as the liquid base ensures that your smoothie is dairy-free and suitable for a plant-based diet.

To boost the nutritional content of your smoothie, consider adding a tablespoon of chia seeds or flaxseeds. These seeds are rich in fiber, omega-3 fatty acids, and protein, which can help keep you full and satisfied until your next meal. For an extra protein punch, you might also add a scoop of plant-based protein powder or a dollop of nut butter.

If you prefer a thicker, more substantial breakfast, opt for a smoothie bowl. To make a smoothie bowl, use less liquid in your blend to achieve a spoonable consistency. Once you have your thick smoothie base, the fun part begins: the toppings. A typical smoothie bowl might be topped with granola for crunch, fresh fruits for added sweetness, and coconut flakes for a tropical twist. A drizzle of nut butter, such as almond or peanut butter, adds a rich, creamy texture and an extra dose of healthy fats and protein. Other popular toppings include chia seeds, hemp seeds, goji berries, and cacao nibs, all of which contribute additional nutrients and flavors.

Smoothies and smoothie bowls are perfect for those on a plant-based diet as they provide a quick and easy way to consume a variety of fruits and vegetables. They ensure you get a good mix of vitamins, minerals, and antioxidants right at the start of your day. Moreover, they can be tailored to meet your specific dietary needs and preferences, whether you're looking to increase your fiber intake, boost your protein levels, or simply enjoy a delicious and nutritious breakfast.

Overnight Oats And Chia Puddings

Overnight oats and chia puddings are the epitome of convenience for plant-based breakfasts, offering a quick and nutritious start to your day with minimal morning effort. Preparing these delicious options the night before ensures you have a ready-to-eat meal waiting for you when you wake up, making them ideal for busy mornings.

Overnight Oats

To make overnight oats, start by combining rolled oats with your preferred plant-based milk. Options like almond, soy, oat, or coconut milk work well. Sweeten the mixture with a touch of maple syrup or agave nectar to enhance the flavor. Next, personalize your oats by adding fruits, nuts, and spices. Popular choices include bananas, berries, chopped nuts, and seeds, along with a pinch of cinnamon or a dash of vanilla extract. Once mixed, transfer the mixture into a jar or a sealed container and refrigerate it overnight. During this time, the oats absorb the liquid, softening and becoming creamy.

Overnight oats are highly customizable, allowing you to tailor them to your taste preferences. For example, you can create a tropical version by adding coconut milk, pineapple chunks, and shredded coconut. Or, opt for a hearty option with almond milk, sliced almonds, and a sprinkle of nutmeg. The possibilities are endless, and experimenting with different combinations can be a fun way to discover your favorite flavor profiles.

Chia Pudding

Chia pudding is another convenient and versatile plant-based breakfast option. To prepare chia pudding, mix chia seeds with your choice of plant-based milk. As the chia seeds soak, they expand and form a gel-like consistency, transforming the mixture into a thick pudding. The basic ratio is generally one part chia seeds to four parts liquid. After mixing, let the pudding sit for at least a few hours or, preferably, overnight in the refrigerator.

To enhance the flavor, consider adding ingredients like cocoa powder, vanilla extract, or fresh fruit. For a chocolate chia pudding, mix in cocoa powder and a sweetener such as maple syrup. Top it with sliced strawberries or raspberries for a delightful treat. Alternatively, a vanilla chia pudding can be made by adding vanilla extract and a touch of agave nectar, topped with fresh berries or mango slices.

Both overnight oats and chia puddings are not only convenient but also packed with nutrients. They provide a good source of fiber, protein, and healthy fats, helping to keep you full and energized throughout the morning. Additionally, the customization options ensure that you can vary your breakfasts to avoid monotony, keeping your meals exciting and flavorful.

Plant-Based Pancakes And Waffles

Who doesn't love a stack of pancakes or a plate of waffles in the morning? The great news is that these breakfast classics can easily be made plant-based without sacrificing taste or texture. Transitioning to plant-based versions of these beloved dishes is simpler than you might think, and the results are just as delicious, if not more so, than their traditional counterparts.

For plant-based pancakes, the key is to substitute traditional dairy milk with plant-based alternatives like almond milk, soy milk, or oat milk. These alternatives provide a creamy base that complements the other ingredients perfectly. Another crucial substitution is the egg replacer. Instead of using eggs, which are a common binding agent in pancake recipes, you can use a flax or chia seed mixture. This mixture is made by combining one tablespoon of ground flax or chia seeds with three tablespoons of water and letting it sit until it becomes gelatinous. This process usually takes about five to ten minutes. The resulting mixture mimics the binding properties of eggs, ensuring your pancakes hold together beautifully.

The rest of the ingredients in plant-based pancakes remain largely the same. You'll need flour, baking powder, a pinch of salt, and a sweetener like maple syrup or agave nectar. The dry ingredients should be mixed in one bowl, while the wet ingredients, including the flax or chia seed mixture, are combined in another. Once both mixtures are ready, they are gently folded together until just combined.

Overmixing can result in tough pancakes, so it's best to mix until the batter is smooth with a few lumps remaining.

Plant-based waffles follow a similar recipe. The primary difference lies in the cooking method, as waffles require a waffle iron to achieve their characteristic crispiness. You can use the same plant-based milk and egg replacer as you would for pancakes. Additionally, you can enhance both pancakes and waffles by adding ingredients like mashed bananas, pumpkin puree, or applesauce. These additions not only provide extra moisture but also infuse your breakfast with delightful flavors and added nutrients.

Topping your plant-based pancakes or waffles is where you can get truly creative. Fresh fruit like berries, bananas, and sliced apples add a burst of natural sweetness and color. Nuts, such as almonds, walnuts, or pecans, provide a satisfying crunch and an extra dose of protein. A drizzle of pure maple syrup or agave nectar completes the dish, adding a touch of indulgence without compromising on nutrition.

Savory Breakfast Options

While sweet breakfasts are delightful, savory options are equally satisfying and offer a nice change of pace. Plant-based diets provide plenty of savory breakfast ideas that are both filling and nutritious.

A popular savory option is the tofu scramble. Tofu, a versatile ingredient, can be crumbled to resemble scrambled eggs in texture. This dish can be flavored with a variety of seasonings to create a rich, eggy taste. Nutritional yeast adds a cheesy flavor and is packed with B vitamins. Turmeric, besides giving a yellow hue reminiscent of eggs, has anti-inflammatory properties. Garlic powder brings a robust taste, and a pinch of black salt, known as kala namak, gives an authentic egg-like flavor due to its sulfur content. To elevate the nutritional profile, you can add an array of vegetables. Spinach is an excellent choice for iron and calcium, tomatoes for their vitamin C and antioxidants, and bell peppers for their vibrant color and crunch, as well as a good dose of vitamins A and C.

Another beloved savory choice is avocado toast. Avocado is a nutrient-dense fruit, rich in healthy monounsaturated fats, fiber, and various vitamins and minerals. Start with a slice of whole-grain toast, which offers a good amount of dietary fiber and complex carbohydrates for sustained energy. Spread mashed avocado generously on the toast, and then let your creativity flow with toppings. Sliced tomatoes add juiciness and a slight tang, while radishes contribute a peppery crunch and a boost of vitamin C. A sprinkle of nutritional yeast can add a cheesy, umami flavor, enhancing the overall taste while providing additional nutrients. To further elevate the flavor, a splash of lemon juice not only brings a refreshing zest but also helps to keep the avocado from browning. A dash of salt and pepper to taste can tie all the flavors together, creating a deliciously balanced breakfast option.

For those looking for more variety, there are numerous other savory plant-based breakfast options. Chickpea flour can be used to make a protein-packed omelet, which can be filled with an assortment of vegetables. Savory oatmeal, made by cooking oats with vegetable broth and adding sautéed vegetables, can be a warm, comforting option. Whole-grain wraps filled with hummus, fresh veggies, and a drizzle of tahini can be a quick, portable breakfast.

Quick And Easy Breakfast Ideas

Mornings can often be the busiest part of the day, making it difficult to prepare a nutritious meal. However, having quick and easy breakfast options can be a real game-changer. These plant-based ideas are not only delicious and healthy but also require minimal preparation, making them perfect for those hectic mornings when you're short on time.

One of the simplest yet satisfying options is fruit and nut butter toast. This versatile breakfast can be customized to suit your taste preferences and dietary needs. Start with a slice of whole-grain toast and spread a generous amount of almond or peanut butter on top. For added flavor and nutrients, top it with sliced bananas, strawberries, or apples. This combination provides a balance of protein, healthy fats, and carbohydrates to keep you energized throughout the morning. Plus, it takes only a few minutes to prepare, making it ideal for those rushed mornings.

Another fantastic option is a breakfast parfait. Parfaits are not only visually appealing but also incredibly easy to make. Take a jar or a glass and layer it with plant-based yogurt, granola, and fresh fruits such as berries, kiwi, or mango. You can prepare these parfaits the night before and store them in the refrigerator, making them a convenient grab-and-go breakfast. The combination of creamy yogurt, crunchy granola, and juicy fruits creates a delightful texture and flavor, ensuring a satisfying start to your day.

Energy bars and bites are also excellent choices for quick breakfasts. These can be made in advance and stored for up to a week, providing a convenient and nutritious option for busy mornings. To make energy bars, blend nuts, seeds, and dried fruits in a food processor until they form a sticky mixture. Press the mixture into a baking dish, refrigerate until firm, and then cut into bars. For energy bites, roll the mixture into small balls. These bars and bites are packed with protein, fiber, and healthy fats, making them a perfect breakfast or snack to fuel your day.

Smoothies are another quick and easy breakfast idea. Blend together your favorite fruits, a handful of spinach or kale, and a plant-based milk or water. For added protein, you can include a scoop of plant-based protein powder or a spoonful of nut butter. Smoothies are highly customizable and can be prepared in advance by portioning out the ingredients in freezer bags. In the morning, simply blend the contents of a bag with your liquid of choice for a nutritious and refreshing breakfast.

CHAPTER FOUR

LUNCH RECIPES

Salads And Grain Bowls

Salads and grain bowls form a cornerstone of plant-based lunches, offering a delightful medley of textures and flavors that cater to individual tastes. These dishes are not only visually appealing but also packed with nutrition, making them a go-to choice for health-conscious eaters.

At the heart of a well-crafted salad or grain bowl lies a base of vibrant leafy greens such as spinach or kale. These greens provide a nutrient-rich foundation, offering essential vitamins and minerals to support overall health. They also contribute a fresh, crisp texture that complements other ingredients beautifully.

Building upon this foundation, a variety of colorful vegetables enhance both the visual appeal and nutritional profile of the dish. Imagine the burst of flavor from juicy cherry tomatoes, the crunch of bell peppers, and the refreshing bite of cucumbers. These vegetables not only add complexity to the dish but also provide a spectrum of vitamins, antioxidants, and dietary fiber.

To elevate the protein content of your salad or grain bowl, consider incorporating ingredients like quinoa, chickpeas, or tofu. Quinoa, a versatile pseudo-grain, offers a complete source of plant-based protein while adding a satisfying chewy texture. Chickpeas, beloved for their nutty flavor and firm texture, are another excellent choice, rich in both protein and fiber. Tofu, with its mild taste and ability to absorb flavors, provides a protein-packed option that complements a variety of seasonings.

No salad or grain bowl is complete without a well-chosen dressing. Whether you prefer a tangy vinaigrette made with citrus juices and olive oil or a creamy tahini dressing blended with garlic and lemon, the dressing ties together the diverse elements of the dish. These dressings not only enhance the flavors but also contribute healthy fats and additional nutrients.

Hearty Soups And Stews

When the weather cools or the craving for comfort strikes, few dishes satisfy quite like hearty soups and stews. These dishes not only warm the body but also nourish with their rich array of flavors and wholesome ingredients. Vegetable-packed soups, such as minestrone or lentil soup, stand out as excellent choices. Brimming with a variety of vegetables, these soups offer a nutritional powerhouse of fiber, vitamins, and minerals essential for maintaining health and vitality.

Minestrone, in particular, delights with its medley of seasonal vegetables—carrots, celery, tomatoes, and beans—simmered to perfection in a savory broth. Its robust flavors are complemented by the heartiness of beans and the subtle sweetness of tomatoes, creating a bowl that's both satisfying and nutritious. Lentil soup, another favorite, brings a hearty dose of protein and fiber, ideal for keeping hunger at bay while supporting digestive health.

For those preferring a more substantial meal, stews provide a comforting alternative. Picture a savory concoction of beans, potatoes, and an assortment of seasonal vegetables, slow-cooked to tender perfection in a flavorful broth. The combination not only satisfies the palate but also offers a wealth of nutrients. Beans, rich in protein and fiber, lend a creamy texture and hearty depth to the stew, while potatoes provide comforting substance.

To round out these meals, consider pairing them with whole grain bread or a side of brown rice. These additions not only enhance the dining experience with their earthy flavors but also contribute complex carbohydrates that sustain energy levels throughout the day. Whether enjoyed as a hearty lunch or a comforting dinner, these soups and stews promise to warm the soul and nourish the body with every spoonful.

Sandwiches And Wraps

Sandwiches and wraps are more than just convenient meals—they're versatile canvases for creating delicious and nutritious lunches. Whether you opt for whole grain bread or a soft wrap, these handheld delights offer endless possibilities to satisfy your palate and keep you fueled throughout the day.

For those seeking a wholesome option, whole grain bread or wraps serve as a sturdy base. They not only provide fiber but also contribute to a satisfying meal that keeps hunger at bay. Layering on ingredients like creamy hummus and nutrient-rich avocado adds both texture and flavor. These additions not only enhance taste but also provide essential fats that are beneficial for heart health.

To boost the nutritional content further, incorporating sliced vegetables such as crisp cucumbers, juicy tomatoes, and crunchy bell peppers adds a burst of freshness. Leafy greens like spinach or arugula not only contribute vitamins and minerals but also lend a delightful crunch. This combination not only enhances the sandwich's taste but also boosts its fiber content, promoting digestive health.

For those craving more protein, consider adding marinated tofu or tempeh. These plant-based proteins offer a satisfying bite and can be grilled to add a smoky flavor. Alternatively, grilled vegetables like zucchini or eggplant provide a hearty, meaty texture without the added animal protein. These options cater to diverse dietary preferences while ensuring a filling meal.

The beauty of sandwiches and wraps lies in their adaptability. They can be tailored to accommodate various dietary needs, from vegetarian to vegan and beyond. For a Mediterranean twist, drizzle with olive oil and sprinkle with herbs like oregano or basil. Adding a squeeze of lemon juice or a dollop of tahini can elevate flavors to new heights.

These handheld meals are perfect for individuals on the go or those looking for a quick yet satisfying lunch option. They can be prepared ahead of time, making them ideal for meal prepping or picnics. Whether enjoyed at work, school, or on a weekend adventure, sandwiches and wraps offer a delicious way to stay nourished throughout the day.

Plant-Based Burgers

Plant-based burgers have surged in popularity, appealing not only to vegans and vegetarians but also to meat-eaters seeking healthier and sustainable alternatives. These burgers are crafted from a variety of plant-based ingredients such as black beans, lentils, quinoa, or mushrooms, meticulously blended to recreate the texture and flavor profile of traditional beef burgers.

What sets plant-based burgers apart is their nutritional profile. They are rich in protein and fiber, thanks to ingredients like black beans and lentils, which provide essential nutrients without the cholesterol and saturated fats found in animal-derived burgers. This makes them a favorable choice for those looking to reduce their intake of meat without compromising on taste or nutrition.

Preparing a plant-based burger involves a creative mix of ingredients. Black beans, for instance, offer a hearty base with a creamy texture, while lentils provide a firmness akin to ground beef. Quinoa adds a nutty flavor and boosts the protein content, making these burgers not only delicious but also satisfyingly filling.

To serve, opt for whole grain buns to enhance the nutritional value with added fiber. Layer the burger with fresh toppings such as crisp lettuce, juicy tomato slices, tangy pickles, and a dollop of vegan mayo or mustard for added zest. This combination not only adds layers of flavor but also contributes to a well-rounded meal that caters to diverse palates.

Plant-based burgers are versatile, allowing for endless variations to suit personal preferences. Some recipes incorporate finely chopped mushrooms to impart a savory umami taste, while others use chickpeas for a creamy consistency. Grilling or pan-searing these burgers enhances their texture, creating a satisfying bite that rivals traditional beef patties.

Beyond their nutritional benefits, plant-based burgers support sustainable food practices by reducing the environmental impact associated with meat production. They require fewer resources like water and land compared to raising livestock, making them a more eco-friendly choice for conscientious consumers.

Lunch On The Go

When life gets hectic and time becomes a precious commodity, having a plan for quick, nutritious lunches is essential. Whether you're rushing between meetings, picking up the kids, or squeezing in a workout, these easy-to-assemble meal ideas ensure you stay fueled and healthy throughout the day.

One of the most versatile and convenient options is a bento box. These compartmentalized containers allow you to pack a variety of foods in one compact package. For a balanced meal, fill your bento box with an assortment of raw vegetables like baby carrots, cherry tomatoes, and cucumber slices. Pair these with fresh fruits such as apple slices, grapes, or berries for a sweet and refreshing touch. Add a handful of nuts and seeds for a crunchy source of healthy fats and protein, ensuring your energy levels stay steady.

Another prep-ahead favorite is the mason jar salad. Layering ingredients in a jar not only keeps them fresh but also makes for an attractive and easy-to-transport meal. Start with a base of leafy greens like spinach or arugula, then add layers of cooked grains such as quinoa or brown rice, followed by protein-rich beans or chickpeas. Top it off with a colorful assortment of chopped vegetables like bell peppers, radishes, and avocado. Seal the jar tightly, and when you're ready to eat, simply shake it up to mix the ingredients and enjoy a satisfying, wholesome meal.

For those who prefer a liquid lunch, smoothies are the ultimate grab-and-go option. Blend together leafy greens like kale or spinach with a mix of fruits such as bananas, strawberries, and mango. Enhance the nutritional value by adding plant-based protein powder or Greek yogurt for creaminess and protein content. Pack your smoothie in a spill-proof container and sip on the go for a refreshing and nutrient-packed lunch.

CHAPTER FIVE

DINNER RECIPES

One-Pot Meals

One-pot meals have become a cornerstone for busy individuals craving convenience without sacrificing flavor. These dishes exemplify culinary ingenuity by harmonizing an array of ingredients into a single cooking vessel, where they meld together to create hearty and satisfying meals.

Picture a bubbling pot of lentil stew, its aroma wafting through the kitchen, promising warmth and nourishment after a long day. Lentils, vegetables, and savory spices gently simmer together, each component contributing to a rich tapestry of flavors. This simplicity in preparation extends beyond just lentils; one-pot meals encompass a diverse range of culinary traditions and ingredients.

Consider a robust chili sin carne, where beans, tomatoes, and spices simmer into a chili that's both hearty and comforting, perfect for gatherings or quiet evenings at home. The slow infusion of flavors transforms basic ingredients into a dish that satisfies both the palate and the soul.

Venture into the realm of paella, where vibrant vegetables, savory rice, and aromatic saffron create a dish that evokes the spirit of Spanish cuisine. In one pot, the rice absorbs the essence of the vegetables and spices, achieving a perfect balance of textures and flavors with every bite.

What makes one-pot meals truly exceptional is their ability to deliver complex flavors with minimal cleanup. By cooking everything in a single pot, from start to finish, these meals streamline the cooking process while maximizing taste. They're not just practical; they're a testament to the art of layering flavors and textures in a way that transforms simple ingredients into extraordinary dishes.

For the busy individual, one-pot meals offer more than just a quick solution; they provide a moment of culinary delight and satisfaction. Whether you're preparing a comforting soup, a fragrant curry, or a hearty risotto, the beauty of one-pot meals lies in their versatility and ability to adapt to different tastes and dietary preferences.

Pasta and noodle dishes epitomize the culinary versatility and creativity found within the plant-based diet. These dishes transcend mere sustenance, offering a canvas where simple ingredients harmonize to create gourmet delights. Imagine a creamy vegan carbonara where cashew cream mimics the richness of traditional dairy, blending seamlessly with al dente spaghetti for a comforting yet guilt-free indulgence. Alternatively, savor the tangy notes of lemon garlic pasta with wilted spinach, a dish that balances freshness and zest in every bite.

The appeal of plant-based pasta and noodle dishes lies not only in their flavor profiles but also in the diversity of textures and ingredients they showcase. Whether it's the chewy satisfaction of udon noodles or the delicate strands of angel hair pasta, each type lends itself uniquely to different culinary interpretations. Fresh herbs like basil or parsley add vibrancy, while vegetables such as roasted cherry tomatoes or sautéed bell peppers contribute both color and nutrients.

Central to these dishes is the integration of plant-based proteins like tofu or tempeh, offering substantial alternatives to meat while enriching flavors and textures. Picture a hearty spaghetti bolognese where crumbled tofu replaces ground beef, simmered in a savory tomato sauce bursting with umami. Such dishes not only satisfy cravings but also support sustainable eating practices, aligning with eco-conscious lifestyles.

Exploring plant-based pasta and noodle dishes is an adventure in discovering how everyday ingredients can transform into culinary masterpieces. Whether you're experimenting with Asian-inspired stir-fries featuring soba noodles and crisp vegetables, or indulging in Mediterranean influences with olive oil, garlic, and sun-dried tomatoes over penne, each dish promises a journey of taste and texture.

Plant-Based Stir-Fries

Stir-fries are the epitome of fast, flavorful cooking in the realm of plant-based cuisine. These dishes marry speed with nutrition, making them beloved staples in kitchens worldwide. Picture this: vibrant vegetables, tofu, or seitan sizzling in a hot pan, infused with aromatic spices and savory sauces. The result? A symphony of colors, textures, and tastes that redefine the art of quick meals.

In the realm of plant-based diets, stir-fries shine brightly for their versatility and health benefits. They offer a perfect canvas for showcasing an array of fresh produce, from crisp bell peppers and tender broccoli florets to earthy mushrooms and delicate snow peas. Tossed together with protein-rich tofu or hearty seitan, these ingredients quickly absorb the flavors of ginger, garlic, soy sauce, and other seasonings, creating a harmony of savory and aromatic notes.

Take, for example, a sesame ginger stir-fry: tender-crisp vegetables lightly caramelized in sesame oil, tossed with marinated tofu and a zesty ginger sauce. Each bite bursts with nutty undertones from sesame seeds, balanced by the freshness of ginger and the umami richness of soy sauce. This dish not only satisfies the palate but also packs a punch of essential nutrients.

For those craving a bolder kick, a spicy Szechuan tofu stir-fry delivers with its fiery blend of Szechuan peppercorns, chili paste, and garlic. The tofu, with its sponge-like ability to soak up flavors, becomes the perfect partner for the intense heat of Szechuan cuisine, tempered by the crunch of water chestnuts and the snap of fresh green beans. This dish is a testament to the adaptability of plant-based ingredients in global cuisines.

Stir-fries not only cater to a spectrum of tastes but also cater to busy schedules. They come together swiftly, making them ideal for weeknight dinners or last-minute meals without compromising on nutrition or taste. Whether you're a seasoned chef or a novice in the kitchen, mastering the art of stir-frying opens doors to a world of culinary creativity and healthful eating.

Casseroles And Bakes

asseroles and bakes embody the essence of comfort and warmth, transforming simple ingredients into hearty, satisfying meals that soothe the soul. These dishes, such as eggplant parmesan or Mexican quinoa casserole, redefine traditional comfort food with innovative, plant-based twists. They're not just meals; they're experiences that bring families and friends together over shared tastes and textures.

At the heart of casseroles and bakes lies their versatility. They're canvases where grains, vegetables, and creamy sauces harmonize beautifully, creating layers of flavor and nourishment. Take, for instance, eggplant parmesan—a classic Italian dish reinvented with tender layers of eggplant, marinara sauce, and vegan cheese, baked to golden perfection. Each bite offers a symphony of savory flavors and a comforting richness that satisfies both palate and spirit.

Similarly, Mexican quinoa casserole bursts with vibrant colors and robust flavors. Quinoa, a protein-packed grain, forms the base, intermingled with black beans, corn, bell peppers, and a medley of spices. Topped with avocado slices and fresh cilantro, it's a celebration of wholesome ingredients that bring the essence of Mexico to the table.

What makes casseroles and bakes particularly appealing is their convenience.

Many recipes allow for make-ahead preparation, perfect for busy weeknights or gatherings where time is precious, yet the desire for wholesome meals remains paramount. Simply assemble the ingredients, layer them in a baking dish, and let the oven work its magic, filling the kitchen with tantalizing aromas that promise a delicious reward.

Beyond their practicality, these dishes often serve as the centerpiece of family gatherings or intimate dinners—a testament to their ability to nourish not just the body but also the bonds that connect us. They evoke memories of home-cooked meals and cherished traditions, offering a taste of familiarity even in the busiest of times.

International cuisine offers a tantalizing array of flavors that are often naturally plant-based or easily adaptable to meet dietary preferences. From the robust spices of Indian curries to the refreshing Mediterranean salads and the umami-rich Japanese sushi rolls, plant-based dishes span the globe, showcasing diverse ingredients and culinary traditions.

In Indian cuisine, dishes like chickpea masala and palak paneer (tofu-based spinach curry) exemplify the vibrant use of spices and legumes. These hearty dishes not only satisfy the palate but also provide essential nutrients. The aromatic blend of spices such as cumin, coriander, and turmeric adds depth to these plant-based delights, making them favorites for vegetarians and vegans alike.

Moving to the Mediterranean, salads take center stage with fresh ingredients like crisp greens, juicy tomatoes, and tangy olives drizzled with olive oil and sprinkled with herbs like oregano and basil. Mediterranean cuisine celebrates simplicity and freshness, creating dishes like falafel wraps filled with chickpea patties, crunchy vegetables, and creamy tahini sauce, all wrapped in warm pita bread.

In Japan, sushi rolls offer a delightful fusion of flavors and textures. Traditional sushi, often featuring vinegared rice, seaweed, and a variety of fresh vegetables like cucumber and avocado, provides a satisfying umami experience without the need for animal products. The artistry and precision in sushi preparation highlight Japan's reverence for food aesthetics and balance.

Italy, renowned for its pasta and risotto, offers comforting plant-based options. Risotto, a creamy rice dish cooked slowly with vegetable broth and often enriched with mushrooms or seasonal vegetables like asparagus or peas, exemplifies Italian culinary finesse. The simplicity of risotto allows the flavors of the ingredients to shine through, creating a satisfying and hearty meal.

Each of these international plant-based dishes not only delights the senses but also underscores the versatility and richness of plant-based ingredients. Whether exploring the spice-laden curries of India, the freshness of Mediterranean salads, the delicate artistry of Japanese sushi, or the comforting allure of Italian risotto, these dishes celebrate the bounty of nature and the art of culinary diversity across cultures.

CHAPTER SIX

SNACKS AND APPETIZERS

Within the realm of plant-based diets, snacks and appetizers assume a pivotal role in maintaining energy levels and satiating cravings throughout the day. These small bites not only serve as quick pick-me-ups but also stand as delightful options for social gatherings. Embracing plant-based ingredients opens up a diverse array of flavors and textures, providing alternatives to conventional snack choices.

For those seeking a nutritious boost, consider options like crispy kale chips seasoned with nutritional yeast for a savory punch or hummus paired with fresh-cut vegetables for a refreshing crunch. These choices not only provide essential nutrients but also cater to varying tastes and dietary preferences.

For a touch of sophistication during gatherings, bruschetta topped with ripe tomatoes, basil, and a drizzle of balsamic glaze can captivate palates while aligning with plant-based principles. Alternatively, stuffed mushrooms filled with quinoa, spinach, and vegan cheese offer a savory bite that satisfies without compromising on flavor.

Plant-based snacks and appetizers showcase the versatility of ingredients such as nuts, seeds, legumes, and whole grains, ensuring a balance of protein, fiber, and essential vitamins. Whether enjoyed solo or shared with others, these plant-powered choices cater to both nutritional needs and culinary enjoyment, proving that plant-based eating can be both satisfying and delicious.

Energy Balls And Bars

Energy balls and bars have emerged as popular choices for those seeking quick, nutrient-packed snacks that deliver sustained energy. These compact treats are crafted from a blend of wholesome ingredients like nuts, seeds, dried fruits, and natural sweeteners such as dates or maple syrup. Their appeal lies not only in their convenience but also in their ability to offer a balanced combination of carbohydrates, healthy fats, and proteins.

At their core, energy balls and bars are designed to provide a quick energy boost without sacrificing nutritional value. Nuts and seeds contribute healthy fats and protein, while dried fruits add natural sweetness and additional nutrients. The use of natural sweeteners like dates or maple syrup ensures these snacks are free from refined sugars, making them a healthier alternative to many store-bought options.

One of the greatest advantages of energy balls and bars is their versatility. They can be easily customized to suit various dietary preferences and flavor profiles. Whether you prefer a chocolatey indulgence, a tangy citrus twist, or a savory nutty blend, there's a recipe to satisfy every craving. Furthermore, they can be adapted to accommodate specific dietary needs such as gluten-free, vegan, or paleo diets, making them inclusive snacks for a wide range of individuals.

Preparing energy balls and bars is remarkably simple and requires minimal culinary skill. Typically, ingredients are blended together in a food processor, rolled into bite-sized balls, or pressed into bars, and then chilled to set. This straightforward process allows for batch preparation, ensuring you always have a stash of nutritious snacks on hand for busy days or post-workout refueling.

In addition to their nutritional benefits and ease of preparation, energy balls and bars are portable and shelf-stable, making them ideal for on-the-go consumption. Whether you're hiking, traveling, or simply need a quick pick-me-up at work, these snacks provide a convenient solution without compromising on quality or taste.

Dips And Spreads

Dips and spreads are invaluable assets in the realm of plant-based snacking, offering both versatility and nutritional benefits. Among the classics, hummus stands tall as a favorite. Crafted from chickpeas, blended with tahini, fresh lemon juice, and a touch of garlic, hummus not only delights the palate but also delivers a robust dose of protein and fiber. This combination makes it a satisfying option for those seeking both flavor and sustenance.

Guacamole, another star in the dips category, boasts a creamy texture and rich flavor derived from ripe avocados, tomatoes, onions, and lime juice. Beyond its delicious taste, guacamole is celebrated for its healthy fats and ample supply of vitamins, making it a wholesome choice for enhancing snacks and meals alike.

Both hummus and guacamole excel as accompaniments to various dishes. They serve as perfect partners for raw vegetables, offering a crunchy contrast that complements their creamy textures. Additionally, they elevate the appeal of whole-grain crackers, transforming a simple snack into a more satisfying and nutritious experience. In sandwiches, these dips shine as spreads, imparting depth of flavor and enriching every bite with their nutritional value.

The appeal of dips and spreads lies not only in their taste but also in their ability to enhance the health profile of snacks and meals. Hummus, with its protein-packed chickpea base, supports muscle health and provides a feeling of fullness, making it an excellent choice for those managing their diet. Guacamole, with its heart-healthy fats and essential vitamins, contributes to overall well-being while satisfying cravings with its creamy texture and tangy undertones.

Plant-Based Finger Foods

Plant-based finger foods are a delightful array of bite-sized treats that cater to both visual appeal and nutritional value. These miniature culinary creations span a diverse spectrum, from crisp vegetable spring rolls to savory stuffed mushrooms and flavorful tofu skewers. Each offering presents a creative opportunity to seamlessly integrate vegetables, legumes, and plant-based proteins into everyday dining, ensuring a satisfying crunch or chew with every bite.

One of the standout features of plant-based finger foods is their versatility. They can be served as appetizers, snacks, or even as part of a main course, adapting effortlessly to various culinary settings. For instance, vegetable spring rolls, with their colorful assortment of fresh veggies wrapped in delicate rice paper, offer a refreshing crunch that complements any dipping sauce, from tangy sweet chili to creamy peanut sauce.

Stuffed mushrooms, another popular choice, combine earthy mushroom caps filled with a medley of ingredients like quinoa, spinach, and vegan cheese, providing a rich umami flavor in a compact package. These can be baked to perfection, enhancing their texture and bringing out their natural flavors.

Tofu skewers, marinated in a blend of spices and herbs before being grilled or baked, offer a protein-packed option that appeals to both vegans and omnivores alike. The tofu absorbs the marinade, creating a flavorful exterior with a tender, chewy center, perfect for dipping into accompanying sauces or enjoying on their own.

What sets plant-based finger foods apart is not just their taste and texture but also their nutritional profile. They are typically low in saturated fats and cholesterol-free, making them a heart-healthy alternative to traditional finger foods. Moreover, they are rich in essential nutrients such as vitamins, minerals, and dietary fiber, contributing to a balanced diet.

Whether you're hosting a gathering, preparing a quick snack, or looking for inventive ways to incorporate more plants into your meals, plant-based finger foods offer a delicious solution. Their appeal lies not only in their vibrant colors and enticing flavors but also in their ability to satisfy cravings while promoting wellness.

Healthy Chips And Crackers

Healthy chips and crackers have become popular alternatives to traditional snacks, offering a crunchy bite without compromising nutritional value. These snacks can be made from a variety of wholesome ingredients, including whole grains, seeds, and vegetables. They provide a delicious way to satisfy cravings while delivering essential nutrients.

One standout option is baked kale chips. Kale, a nutrient-dense leafy green, is rich in vitamins A, C, and K, which are crucial for maintaining healthy skin, boosting the immune system, and supporting blood clotting and bone health. To make kale chips, simply tear kale leaves into bite-sized pieces, toss them in olive oil, and sprinkle with sea salt. Bake until crispy, and you have a snack that is not only delicious but also packed with antioxidants and other beneficial compounds.

Whole-grain crackers are another excellent choice for healthy snacking. These can be made from a variety of grains, such as oats, quinoa, or brown rice, all of which offer a good source of fiber and complex carbohydrates. Fiber is essential for digestive health, helping to regulate bowel movements and prevent constipation, while complex carbohydrates provide a steady release of energy, keeping you fuller for longer. Whole grains also contain a range of vitamins and minerals, including B vitamins, iron, and magnesium, which support energy production and overall health.

Flaxseed crackers are a popular seed-based snack. Flaxseeds are high in omega-3 fatty acids, which are known for their anti-inflammatory properties and role in supporting heart health. These crackers are easy to make at home by combining ground flaxseeds with water and seasoning them with herbs and spices before baking. The result is a crispy, flavorful snack that contributes to your daily intake of healthy fats and fiber.

Vegetable-based chips, such as sweet potato or beet chips, offer another nutritious alternative to traditional potato chips. Sweet potatoes are rich in beta-carotene, a precursor to vitamin A, which supports vision and immune function. Beets are high in nitrates, which can help improve blood flow and lower blood pressure. Both vegetables provide a good source of dietary fiber and can be baked or air-fried to create a crunchy, satisfying snack.

Homemade healthy chips and crackers allow you to control the ingredients and avoid additives and preservatives often found in store-bought versions. Experimenting with different seasonings, such as garlic powder, paprika, or nutritional yeast, can add variety and enhance the flavor of your snacks.

Sweet And Savory Snacks

When it comes to plant-based snacking, the options are both diverse and delicious, catering to a wide range of taste preferences. Whether you're in the mood for something sweet or craving a savory bite, plant-based snacks provide a wholesome and satisfying option. Here's a deeper dive into some delightful sweet and savory plant-based snacks that not only tantalize your taste buds but also align with a healthy lifestyle.

Sweet Treats

For those with a sweet tooth, plant-based snacks can be both indulgent and nutritious. One delightful option is fruit skewers drizzled with dark chocolate. This snack combines the natural sweetness of fresh fruits with the rich, slightly bitter flavor of dark chocolate. You can use a variety of fruits such as strawberries, pineapple, and banana slices, which are threaded onto skewers and then drizzled with melted dark chocolate. Not only do these skewers look appealing, but they also provide a burst of vitamins, antioxidants, and fiber, making them a healthy yet satisfying treat.

Another fantastic sweet snack is homemade fruit sorbet. This refreshing dessert is made by blending frozen berries with coconut milk. Berries like strawberries, blueberries, and raspberries are packed with antioxidants and vitamins, while coconut milk adds a creamy texture and a hint of tropical flavor. This sorbet is not only easy to prepare but also free from added sugars and artificial ingredients, making it a guilt-free indulgence. It's perfect for hot days or as a light dessert after a meal.

Savory Options

If you're in the mood for something savory, roasted chickpeas are an excellent choice. Chickpeas, also known as garbanzo beans, are a fantastic source of plant-based protein and fiber. To make roasted chickpeas, simply toss cooked chickpeas with olive oil, and your favorite herbs and spices, and bake them until they are crispy. Seasonings can vary from smoked paprika and cumin for a smoky flavor to garlic and rosemary for a more aromatic taste. These crunchy delights are not only delicious but also incredibly nutritious, providing a satisfying crunch that's perfect for snacking.

Seaweed snacks are another savory option that is both tasty and nutritious. Seaweed is rich in minerals like iodine, which is essential for thyroid function, as well as vitamins A, C, and E. These snacks are typically made by roasting seaweed sheets until they are crispy and then lightly seasoning them with sea salt or other flavors. The result is a light, crispy snack that is low in calories but high in nutritional value.

CHAPTER SEVEN

DESSERTS

Plant-Based Cakes And Cupcakes

Cakes and cupcakes often serve as the centerpiece of celebrations, from birthdays to weddings, and plant-based versions can be just as impressive and delectable as their traditional counterparts. The key to crafting a great plant-based cake or cupcake lies in using ingredients that effectively replace traditional dairy and eggs without compromising on taste or texture. Fortunately, there are numerous options available to achieve this.

One of the most popular substitutes for dairy milk in plant-based baking is almond milk, which has a slightly nutty flavor that pairs well with many types of cake. Soy milk is another excellent option, known for its creamy consistency and neutral taste. Coconut milk, with its rich and unique flavor, can also add an exotic twist to your baked goods. When it comes to replacing eggs, flaxseeds or chia seeds mixed with water are common alternatives. These mixtures form a gel-like consistency that mimics the binding properties of eggs.

Classic cake flavors such as vanilla, chocolate, and red velvet can be easily adapted to plant-based recipes. For instance, a vegan chocolate cake can be made using cocoa powder, coconut oil, and plant-based milk. Incorporating a bit of apple cider vinegar into the batter helps the cake rise and contributes to a moist, fluffy texture. This is because the vinegar reacts with baking soda, creating bubbles that expand during baking.

The art of plant-based baking extends beyond the cake itself to the frosting. Traditional frostings, which typically rely on butter and cream, can be transformed into delicious plant-based versions. For a classic buttercream, plant-based butter made from ingredients like coconut oil or sunflower oil can be used. Powdered sugar remains a staple, and natural flavorings such as vanilla extract, lemon zest, or even espresso can be added to enhance the taste. For a richer, more indulgent option, consider using coconut cream, which whips up beautifully and adds a luscious texture.

In addition to these basic ingredients, experimenting with other plant-based components can lead to delightful variations. For example, mashed bananas or applesauce can add moisture and sweetness, while avocado can be used for its creamy texture and healthy fats. Nut butters, such as almond or cashew, can introduce a new dimension of flavor and richness to both cakes and frostings.

Plant-based baking is not just about substituting ingredients; it's also about embracing creativity and exploring new flavors and textures. With the right ingredients and techniques, you can create plant-based cakes and cupcakes that are every bit as delicious and satisfying as traditional versions. Whether you're baking for a special occasion or simply indulging your sweet tooth, these plant-based treats are sure to impress both vegans and non-vegans alike.

Cookies and bars are perfect for satisfying sweet cravings in a more portable form. Plant-based cookies can be made with a variety of flours, such as almond flour, oat flour, or whole wheat flour. These flours not only provide a different texture and flavor but also contribute to the nutritional profile of the cookies. For instance, almond flour is rich in protein and healthy fats, while oat flour is high in fiber and whole wheat flour offers a good balance of nutrients. Natural sweeteners like maple syrup, agave nectar, or coconut sugar can replace refined sugars, providing a healthier twist without compromising taste. These sweeteners are less processed and often come with additional nutrients, making them a better option for health-conscious bakers.

For chocolate chip cookies, using dark chocolate chips or chunks that are dairy-free is a great way to keep them plant-based. Dark chocolate has a higher cocoa content and is typically lower in sugar than milk chocolate, offering a richer flavor. Additionally, it contains antioxidants and can be beneficial in moderation. Adding nuts, seeds, or dried fruits can enhance the texture and flavor of your cookies. Nuts like walnuts, almonds, or pecans provide a satisfying crunch and additional protein and healthy fats. Seeds such as chia, flax, or sunflower add a unique texture and are packed with nutrients like omega-3 fatty acids and fiber. Dried fruits, such as cranberries, raisins, or apricots, introduce natural sweetness and chewiness, along with vitamins and minerals.

Bars, such as granola bars or brownies, can also be made plant-based. Using ingredients like oats, nuts, dates, and cocoa powder, you can create bars that are not only delicious but also packed with nutrients. Oats are a fantastic base for granola bars, offering a hearty texture and a good source of fiber. Combining them with nuts and seeds provides a satisfying crunch and boosts the protein and healthy fat content. Dates serve as a natural sweetener and binder, adding a caramel-like flavor and sticky texture that helps hold the bars together. Cocoa powder can be used to make chocolate-flavored bars, providing a rich taste and additional antioxidants.

To make these bars, you can start by mixing rolled oats, chopped nuts, and seeds in a bowl. In a separate bowl, blend pitted dates until smooth, then mix them with the dry ingredients. Add a touch of maple syrup or agave nectar for additional sweetness if desired. Press the mixture firmly into a baking dish and refrigerate until set. For a chocolate twist, add cocoa powder to the mix or melt dairy-free dark chocolate to drizzle on top.

Pies And Tarts

Pies and tarts, classic comfort foods, can easily be transformed into plant-based delights with a few thoughtful substitutions. Whether it's a flaky pie crust or a rich tart shell, plant-based alternatives for crusts and fillings can deliver both taste and texture.

Crust Options

A traditional pie crust often relies on butter and refined flour, but plant-based versions can be equally delicious and versatile. Almond flour and oat flour are excellent choices for a gluten-free and nutrient-dense base. These flours provide a subtle nutty flavor that pairs well with a variety of fillings. Crushed nuts and dates offer another creative option. By blending nuts like almonds or walnuts with soft, sweet dates, you can create a crust that is both chewy and flavorful. This type of crust doesn't require baking, making it perfect for raw tarts or quick pie recipes.

To bind the crust, coconut oil or plant-based butter can be used. Coconut oil, with its mild sweetness, works well in both sweet and savory applications, while plant-based butter can replicate the rich, buttery flavor of traditional crusts. Simply combine your chosen flour or nut mixture with the binding agent and press it into a pie pan or tart tin. Pre-bake if necessary, or chill to set.

Filling Options

When it comes to fillings, fruits are a natural and delicious choice. Classic options like apple pie, berry tart, and pumpkin pie can all be made plant-based with minimal adjustments. Fresh or frozen fruits can be sweetened with natural sugars like maple syrup or agave, and thickened with cornstarch or arrowroot powder to achieve the right consistency.

For creamy fillings, a mixture of blended silken tofu, cashews, or coconut cream can mimic traditional dairy-based ones. Silken tofu, when blended, has a smooth, custard-like texture that works wonderfully in pies like pumpkin or chocolate mousse. Cashews, soaked and blended, create a rich, creamy base that can be flavored to suit any tart filling. Coconut cream, with its natural sweetness and thick consistency, is perfect for tropical flavors or as a whipped topping.

Spices and flavorings play a crucial role in enhancing plant-based pies and tarts. Cinnamon, nutmeg, and vanilla extract are classic additions that can bring warmth and depth to your desserts. These spices complement the natural flavors of fruits and creamy fillings, making each bite as comforting as traditional versions.

Frozen Treats

Frozen treats are an excellent way to cool down on a hot day or satisfy a craving for something sweet and refreshing. In the realm of plant-based diets, frozen desserts can be both delicious and nutritious, using alternatives like coconut milk, almond milk, or soy milk as bases. These options provide a creamy texture and rich flavor without the need for dairy.

One of the simplest and most delightful plant-based frozen desserts is banana ice cream, often referred to as "nice cream." To make this, blend frozen bananas until they reach a smooth, creamy consistency. This base can be customized with various flavors and add-ins. For a chocolatey treat, add a tablespoon of cocoa powder or a handful of vegan chocolate chips. For a classic vanilla taste, a splash of vanilla extract works wonders. Fresh or frozen berries can also be blended in for a fruity twist, making this treat versatile and endlessly customizable. The natural sweetness of bananas eliminates the need for added sugars, making it a healthier option.

Another fantastic plant-based frozen treat is sorbet. Sorbet is primarily made from fruit puree and a bit of sweetener, making it naturally plant-based and incredibly refreshing. The beauty of sorbet lies in its simplicity and the vibrant flavors it offers. To make a basic sorbet, choose your favorite fruits—mango, pineapple, and berries are popular choices. Blend the fruit into a smooth puree, and if needed, add a sweetener like agave syrup or maple syrup to enhance the flavor. The puree is then frozen, resulting in a refreshing and flavorful treat.

For a more complex flavor profile, consider combining different fruits. For example, a mango-pineapple sorbet offers a tropical taste that's perfect for summer. A berry blend, combining strawberries, blueberries, and raspberries, provides a burst of flavor with every bite. Experimenting with different combinations can lead to exciting new flavors and ensure that your frozen treats are always interesting.

Additionally, you can create frozen popsicles using plant-based ingredients. Mix fruit juices with pieces of fresh fruit and pour them into popsicle molds. Coconut water with chunks of kiwi and strawberries makes for a hydrating and delicious popsicle. For a creamier option, blend coconut milk with mango puree and freeze in molds.

For those who want to enjoy dessert while keeping it on the healthier side, there are plenty of plant-based options that are both delicious and nutritious. These options not only satisfy your sweet tooth but also provide essential nutrients, making them a perfect choice for a health-conscious diet.

Chia Pudding

One of the most popular healthy dessert options is chia pudding. Chia seeds are packed with fiber, omega-3 fatty acids, and protein, making them a nutritious addition to your diet. To make chia pudding, simply mix chia seeds with plant-based milk such as almond, soy, or coconut milk. The general ratio is about three tablespoons of chia seeds to one cup of milk. Let this mixture sit overnight in the refrigerator. By the next morning, the chia seeds will have absorbed the liquid and expanded, creating a pudding-like texture. You can customize chia pudding by adding flavors like vanilla extract, cocoa powder, or mashed fruits. Top it with fresh berries, sliced bananas, or a drizzle of maple syrup for added sweetness and flavor.

Fruit-Based Desserts

Fruit-based desserts are another excellent option for a healthy treat. Fruits are naturally sweet and full of vitamins, minerals, and antioxidants. One simple and delicious option is baked apples. Core the apples and place them in a baking dish.

Sprinkle them with cinnamon and a touch of maple syrup or agave nectar. Bake at 350°F (175°C) for about 20-25 minutes until the apples are tender. The warmth of the baked apples combined with the aromatic cinnamon and natural sweetness creates a comforting dessert that feels indulgent without being unhealthy.

Fruit Salads

Another delightful way to enjoy fruits is by making fruit salads. Start with a mix of your favorite fresh, seasonal fruits. Berries, melons, citrus fruits, and tropical fruits like mango and pineapple work well together. To enhance the flavors, you can add a drizzle of agave nectar or a splash of freshly squeezed lemon or lime juice. For a bit of crunch, sprinkle some chopped nuts like almonds, walnuts, or pecans on top. You can also add a handful of seeds, such as pumpkin or sunflower seeds, for extra texture and nutrition.

Frozen Banana Bites

For a fun and easy dessert, try making frozen banana bites. Slice a banana into bite-sized pieces, dip them in melted dark chocolate, and place them on a baking sheet lined with parchment paper. Freeze until the chocolate is firm. These bites are not only delicious but also provide a good source of potassium and antioxidants.

Smoothie Bowls

Smoothie bowls are another versatile and healthy dessert option. Blend frozen fruits like berries, bananas, and mangoes with a splash of plant-based milk until smooth. Pour the smoothie into a bowl and top with your favorite toppings such as granola, shredded coconut, fresh fruit, and chia seeds. Smoothie bowls are refreshing, nutrient-dense, and can be customized to suit your taste preferences.

THE END

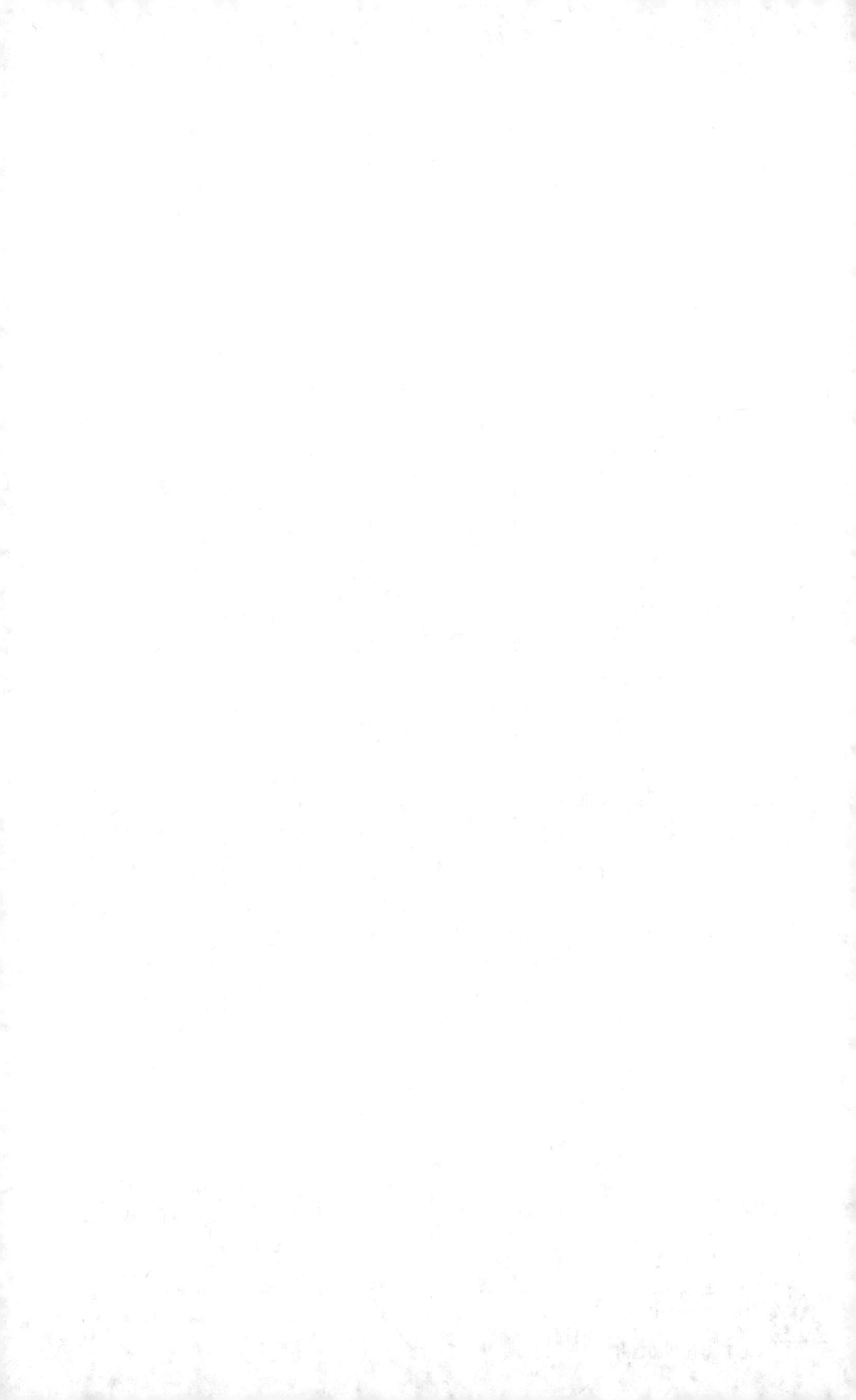